GUIDED MEDITATION

Several meditations for you to relax and become mindful

Lesley Graham

CONTENTS

GUIDED MEDITATION AND MINDFULNESS

Mindfulness is about observation without criticism, being kind and compassionate with yourself. When stress or unhappiness hover overhead, rather than taking it all personally, you learn to treat them as if they were black clouds in the sky and you learn to observe them with curiosity as they float by.

Guided Meditation is simply meditation with the help of a guide. It is one of the easiest ways to enter into a state of deep relaxation and inner stillness. It is one of the most powerful ways to eliminate stress and bring about positive personal changes within yourself.

As the brain does not distinguish between an imagined event and a real one, the experience you have with a guided meditation is just like having a real experience. This has an amazing effect on your life due to the way the brain works.

While you are in this deeply relaxed state of mind, your subconscious is open to positive suggestions, and your guide will use this time to take you on an inner journey that is designed to improve one or more aspects of your life.

I am hoping that reading my Guided Meditations you will benefit from imagining you are doing something else or you are somewhere else.

It enables you to switch off from your anxieties and problems for a few mins and helps you to calm down and relax.

The brain will quite often come back to your problems but this is quite normal and what the brain does. You can very gently bring your attention back to the guided imagery meditation.

Less than 10 minutes of hypnotic guided meditation can reduce stress and blood pressure.

I hope you enjoy these short and pleasant guided meditations and you can read them any time during the day or night.

THE WHITE HORSE

Relax and make yourself really comfortable, take a few deep breaths before we start our Guided Meditation.

Imagine you are going for a nice evening stroll in to the countryside in late summer when the evening is long and warm and the heat from the sun during the day is still in the air and on the ground. You have light and comfortable clothes and shoes on.

You walk and walk and enjoy every step of the way. One of the real joys of summer is to make more of the summer evenings and getting yourself out on foot. You feel relaxed and very comfortable.

You are walking through a meadow which is rich in wildflowers, a host of wildlife providing courtship displays and nesting. There is an abundance of pollinating insects including bees. You are surrounded by this beauty and you are feeling really good. You continue to walk until you come to a style which you have to climb over.

By now it is getting slightly darker and the sun has started to set. The sky takes on shades of orange, the colour that gives you hope that the sun will set only to rise again tomorrow.

You start to climb over the style and jump in to the next field. This field has a lot of trees in it so is looking much darker and the sun is fading only to be replaced by a stunning bright moon. You see the bright light of the moon reflecting beautifully over your skin. Just as the sun has healing energy, so does the moon. You decide to lie down and bathe in the full moons healing light. You close your eyes for a few moments, and when you open them again you see in the distance a brilliant white, the most stunning horse looking at you. He stands still and silent. You can not

Believe your eyes! This beautiful creature slowly starts to walk towards you. You stand perfectly still so as not to frighten him away. He is the most beautiful horse you have ever seen. He eventually comes walking over to you and starts to rub his head against you as if you say Hello. He is so very friendly but has an air of loneliness about him. The horse is alone and you are alone too. He bends down for you and allows you to climb on to his back, you manage to get on to this lovely horse and he very gently starts to stand up for you. You feel very safe and feel that the horse is looking after you and is here for a reason. He turns back around and walks very slowly to get you used to him. You won't fall off and anyway is he looking after you.

He continues to walk. You have no idea at all where he is taking you to. You discover that the horse is life itself, a metaphor but also an example of life's mystery and unpredictability.

This beautiful white shiny horse starts to trot and you are still feeling very safe, but before you know it, he starts to gallop. You gallop and you feel almost at one with this magical white horse that literally came out of nowhere!

He gallops faster and faster and you manage to hold on to him and you feel totally invigorated by the ride, your hair is flying all over and the moonlight is catching all the movements of the horse. He is captivating with the light on every muscle and his white mane turns to silver in this moonlight. You simply cannot take your eyes off such beauty. Your problems and anxiety have disappeared altogether.

He turns in to another field and slows down as he approaches a very deep but still lake. You can't even see a ripple from the water but you can see the moonlight reflecting on the still motionless water. The lovely horse edges closer and closer towards the lake. The moonlight seems to get bigger and bigger as you get nearer to the edge. The skies are full of stars and the moonlight on this horse is stunning.

The horse very gently bends down to allow you to jump off his back and you stand for a moment or two mesmerized by the silence and stillness of the water. The water is still warm from the hot summers day and you take your shoes off and sit down on the very edge of the lake and dip your toes in to it. The warmth immediately relaxes you and makes you feel sleepy. You look up for a moment and notice your own reflection in the lake and the white horse is standing directly behind you. You both have a reflection in the lake. It is like a mirror it is so still.

It dawns on you at that moment that all your problems back home are so small, your anxiety has gone, depression and worries don't really exist. Your mind and brain have been tormenting you for months. Your brain produces thoughts all the time but you don't have to believe them. They are only thoughts! Not fact.

The horse seems to look at you with a knowing, he knows what your worries have been and he is trying to show you that this simple lake and moonlight which costs nothing at all and is free is the most beautiful thing you have experienced in a long time. Its magical! The horse is magical and it's a dream. You have escaped your thoughts for a while. You can escape your thoughts every time you allow yourself to go somewhere else in your mind. Nothing in your mind is ever as bad as it seems and if you can escape for a few mins you will look back and realise this. Try and create space between you and your thoughts so that you can react more calmly and allows you to catch negative thought patterns before they tip you down in a downward spiral. It begins the process of putting you back in control. You have learned something very special this evening and you feel like you are back in control. The lovely white horse bends down again for you to climb back on to his back. He gallops off at great speed with you feeling marvellous and you can't thank him enough for bringing you back down to earth again. He takes you straight back to where you found him and allows you to climb off him. You both stare at each other for a while and he turns around and trots off. You look for him in the dark but he has gone.

You turn around and go back over that style and back across the fields and take yourself off home.

You have to ask yourself was that a dream? Was it real? But it made You switch off from yourself for a while.

Remember Life is 10% what happens to you and 90% how you react to it.

A WALK TO THE BEACH AT SUNRISE

Relax and make yourself really comfortable. Breathe deeply, exhale and let's start our journey.

It's very early in the morning and you are going for a nice peaceful walk on a lovely peaceful beach. In the morning just before sunrise. The sunrise is far superior to the sunset as it is loaded with fresh promise and endless potential.

You are walking along an empty beach, nobody is around yet as it is so early. The sun has not even started to rise yet. You walk and walk for quite a long distance and you are beginning to unwind and relax and are feeling really good about things and yourself.

As you continue to walk further you come across some beautiful little beach huts all in a row. You walk along and can't help noticing how they all look so alike, like little boxes of candy. They are all painted in stripes, and all different colours. They look so lovely and remind you of summertime. As you walk along the row of beach huts you reach the end of the row and you gasp as you see a magnificent beach hut, it is so beautiful! It has duck egg blue clapboard exterior which brings a special rustic charm. It even has a salt-weathered veranda. Little flowers and hanging baskets are all around this charming little hut. You promptly go in to your pocket and bring out a key, and you put it in the lock and the door opens. This lovely little beach hut belongs to you. The inside is just as beautiful as the outside with its stripped floors and white washed walls. It has absolutely everything that you need inside. You decide to make yourself a well-earned cup of tea and you pull up a rocking chair and snuggle up under a blanket on the veranda.

You notice that the sun is starting to rise and a ribbon of tangerine catches your eyes. The sky has become salmon pink and you sit from your veranda and stare at this for a while. You also are aware that the tide has changed and is starting to come in. You see an expanse of wet sand just waiting for the sea to come in and take it all away.

You get up from your rocking chair and walk down to the sea. You search for a stick and start writing thoughts in to this wet sand. You write ANXIETY, DEPRESSION, WORRIES, FEAR, DOUBT. You write all the things down which are a concern to you or are causing you anxiety. You throw the stick back in to the sea and start to walk back to your beach hut.

You sit back on your rocking chair and pull the blanket around you and close your eyes for a few moments.

After a while you open your eyes after resting and you are feeling much more relaxed. You look out to the sea and notice that the sea has completely covered up all your words and they have disappeared forever. The sea and tide swept them all away.

No more worries and no more anxiety no more going over the same stuff in your head. It's all been washed away by the tide.

You now see people walking about and the little cafe and ice cream parlours are all open and ready for business. The sun is much higher in the sky now and you feel it is time to head off home. You fold up your blanket and wash your tea cup up and put your rocking chair back inside off the veranda.

You lock the door of your beach hut. You very quietly say thank you to your beach hut for allowing you to feel peace and calmness again. Your little bit of paradise!
You walk home now and get on with the rest of your day.
You are relaxed and more focused now.

SPRING TIME

Relax and make yourself very comfortable, take a few deep breaths and I shall make you feel more relaxed with this guided meditation.

Imagine yourself walking through a meadow in Spring time, when the sun is warming up and everything is starting to blossom. You are walking in to a spectacular scene. The meadow is home to a rich tapestry of wildlife.

As you continue further you find yourself walking under deciduous trees where a sea of English bluebells rekindles memories of springtime woodland walks, when the days start to lengthen and the weather starts to warm up. You are in awe of this beautiful sight.

The nodding violet blue flowers around your feet where ever you tread. These hardy native bulbs are attracting insects to their delicately scented flowers.

You are becoming very relaxed now as you walk further and further. These vigorous beauties form a dense carpet of spring colour.

You turn around from under the trees and become aware of a beautiful spring meadow. It is so beautiful that it almost takes your breath away! You decide to sit down and look across a sea of grasses swaying back and forth in the cool wind which is gently blowing through the whole meadow. You put your hand out to touch the grasses. The grasses are never static and they create a wonderful feeling of motion. Their graceful motion catches the sunlight. They make you feel wonderful and relaxed.

You stand up once more and continue to walk through the meadow being careful not to tread on the flowers. You take your shoes off and feel the earth and grass beneath your feet. You feel so free and happy that you start to skip and dance through the sea of flowers. You are light and free. You are no longer burden down with problems and worries. As you walk your way across the meadow you spot a Common Spotted Orchid, this delicate flower spreads across your meadowland in pinks and whites. You bend down and take a closer look at their beautiful blotchy leaves.

You love this feeling beneath your feet and you become aware of the Marble White butterflies with their striking black and white mosaic patterned wings. How they flutter and fly in and out of the long grasses and around your face and hair.

You hear a sound and you stop to look for it, you follow the sound and you see a Meadow Grasshopper hanging from a stork. You smile at him. This has been a fantastic experience for you today in this beautiful meadow. You sit amongst the Cowslips with their tube-like egg yolk yellow flowers all clustered together at the end of tall green stems.

You now feel quite tired after your long walk and all that dancing and skipping through the grasses, so you decide to walk back now

You walk back home feeling like your walk has taken your anxieties away and has allowed you to escape for a little while.

You can come back to the spring meadow whenever you wish to experience the beauty and sounds of the meadow,

INNER PEACE BEGINS THE MOMENT YOU CHOOSE NOT TO ALLOW ANOTHER PERSON OR EVENT TO CONTROL YOUR EMOTIONS.

REMOTE ISLAND

Relax and make yourself really comfortable. Imagine yourself on a remote island, you have it all to yourself and nobody else lives there. You are completely surrounded by the sea water. The sound of the waves is such a calming sound. You can take anyone along with you to this quiet and remote place, you could take your partner, friend, someone who is no longer here, a pet, even an actor or actress from your favourite film. You may choose to be alone, after all it's your island so you can choose.

It is so peaceful here and you can let go of all your worries and problems. Nobody or anything can hurt you here.

The trees are blowing and you can hear their soft sound all the time calming and soothing you.

You see birds fly over to the island and seagulls frequently come in.

Imagine what you could do here with so much free time. You could read a book or learn a new language or play sports. I want you to imagine what you would do here on this remote island with its gentle breeze and rhythmic sounding waves.

I would say that life on an island teaches us to be patient because they happen at their own pace. You would have to find water and food, what sort of shelter would you create? It's not a 5-star resort!

Would you enjoy the powdery sand and deepening shades of turquoise on this idyllic patch of paradise?

You are miles from anywhere and you don't even have a boat to take you shopping or to see friend or family. What if you got poorly or frightened?

It's everyone's dream to be on a remote island, miles from anywhere. But is it what's it cracked up to be?

We think we have so many problems and we worry constantly about money, relationships, illness and we could suffer with depression or stress. We think by living on an island would take all that away but how would we feel without family or friends to talk and help us. We have church's everywhere, there won't be a church on an island. We have Doctors and hospitals. We have our children and partners here. On the island there would be no shops or hairdressers. No purpose to our life at all except to survive. To eat and drink!

Maybe our problems don't seem so bad now as we have everything that we need right here where we live. The phone to call anyone at any time, computers, cars and vehicles parked outside our homes. We have it really easy when you think of how difficult it would be on that remote island in the sun. A couple of days in the sunshine and bathing and paddling in the blue sea we would soon bore and tire of.

I think trying to live on a deserted island would be almost impossible, could you catch your lunch every day from the sea? could you survive on coconuts? What about monkeys and snakes at night! Sleeping outdoors in a hammock.

NO THANK YOU

You now feel like your anxieties and problems are not so bad and you feel relieved that you have the life you have.
It's not so bad is it?

THE RAIN FOREST

Imagine you are in a rainforest, miles away from home. This will be a truly exceptional experience. You are in this rainforest a tall dense jungle. You start to walk through this rainforest and the first thing that you notice is the humid heat which is so different to anything that you have experienced before.

It occurs to you that as many as 30 million species of plants and animals live in this rainforest. What a thought! You continue to walk and you become aware of the lush and humid stretches of land covered in tall, broadleaf evergreen trees. You become very relaxed as you take it slowly and you have a long day here and you plan to spend one night here also. You are very excited at this. The temperature has reached around 86 degrees Fahrenheit and you are becoming very warm.

You look up and see a canopy of trees. This area is comprised of the tops of the trees and vines, you cannot believe how large this area is. You look further down and you see ferns and flowers and tree trunks, dead leaves are absolutely everywhere. Where ever you tread you can hear the crunch of them under your feet. You like to hear this and it make you smile!

After a while the heat and humidity and lack of wind makes you feel very tired indeed. You look ahead and notice a river, you become excited by this and you walk up to the gentle flowing water and get in it to cool off for a while. You feel whole again and full of energy once more. You spend the day picking up coconuts and eating whatever fruit you recognise. You have also brought a rucksack with you which you carry on your back. In this you have fresh water and food for the day and a few snacks for tonight. You have walked for quite a long distance by now and your anxiety and stress has completely gone whilst you concentrate on this rainforest experience.

You can hear the woodpeckers in the canopy of trees above you and see monkeys and flying squirrels. You can hear the sound of the high-pitched screech of a million bugs!

The day is soon coming to an end and you have to prepare yourself for this evening. You manage to find a nice spot near the river where you construct a very basic and simple construction from tree trunks and canvas that you have in your rucksack. You get yourself together whilst having a snack and some cool fresh water. You sit for a while and watch the river. This river is flowing slowly over boulders and rocks and trees which have fallen in to it. You watch this for a while and find it soothing and relaxing.

You put a blanket in to your little hut and lay down to try and settle for the night. You suddenly become very aware of the crickets and frogs. What an experience and you love it! Squeals and croaking everywhere.

Then quite suddenly a rainstorm comes in, there is nothing quite like going to sleep at night with a tropical rainstorm pouring down huge drops of water on your little hut. After the hot day, the relative cool that accompanies the rain and the sounds of the drops are mesmerising. It is a simple pleasure that cannot be compared, as you pull your thin sheet over you to fend off the damp cool that filters in through the screens of your little hut.

You feel like you are at the end of the world and feel quite isolated even though the animals never stop all night long.

You survived the night! It was noisy and you could hear the water from the river.

You have really loved your time here in the rainforest and you have learned that you can escape from your thoughts and your mind and your worries. You have control over your thoughts. Unlike the rainforest that has no control over itself with its constant growing of trees and animals screeching constantly and the rain which falls all the time over and over again.

BEN NEVIS

Make yourself really comfortable before I begin this guided meditation.

Imagine you are going on a mountain walk, walking on the highest mountain in the British Isles, Ben Nevis. Standing at 1,345 metres above sea level, it is at the western end of the Grampian Mountains in the Lochaber area of the Scottish Highland. Very close to the town of Fort William.

You are wrapped up in all the right clothes and good solid boots. You are feeling very calm and very relaxed. In all its profound beauty this is a chance of a lifetime. You start your walk and know that it is around 4 miles each way, there and back, quite a challenge!

There is a footpath which you can follow and you start to climb very slowly at first until you get used to it. You are amazed how you are able to climb with such ease. The weather is being kind to you at the moment. When you look to the peaks at the top, they are absolutely stunning with soft fluffy snow on them.

The path is relatively easy to follow but you also have your map with you. You keep following the same route until it seems to flatten out a bit and gives you time to catch your breath.

After walking for quite a long time you reach a beautiful lake and it is covered in a thick mountain mist. The path is becoming a little rockier in places so you need to watch your footing. You then have to cross a small waterfall which you found easy. When it's been raining this waterfall will be much heavier.

You are thoroughly enjoying this challenge and calms your racing mind down. Your worries simply do not exist here. They seem a lifetime away.

You are aware of other hikers doing the same journey and path as you. As you climb higher and higher you notice that the weather is closing in on you a little with little white snowflakes starting to fall. How stunning and beautiful they look. You feel quite safe as you can still see other people and you can hear them happily chatting away.

More than anything you want to reach the summit, you feel that if you can manage this then nothing else in your life could ever be or seem as difficult.

You keep climbing using the steps conveniently provided. You notice that after the first initial steepness, the path does even out to a more moderate slog. The path is very well trodden.

The low clouds are all around you now and it is beginning to snow even harder. You feel tired but exhilarated at the same time.

What a fantastic job you are doing and you feel like you have really achieved something so special and could never ever imagine yourself doing this. You stop for a while and have a cup of tea from your flask and a couple of sandwiches. They do taste good and the tea warms you up as you are beginning to feel quite cold now. As you get higher and higher you really can feel the chill from the heavy snow and blustery winds which have just started at that point.

You have been climbing for a few hours now and have almost reached the summit of Ben Nevis, it is a product of a long extinct volcano and comprises of a large stony plateau of about 100 acres with a large, solidly built cairn approximately 10 feet high.

Well you made it! You have done it and reached the top of this very tall and dangerous mountain.

The view at the top was worth everything that you suffered on the way up. The legendary peak towers above glistening lochans and deep glacial valleys. You realise that in Scotland you can't get any higher than this!

You feel so proud of yourself for managing this very difficult challenge.

You conquered the mountain, so you can now conquer yourself!

Try and live your life each day as you would climb a mountain. An occasional glance towards the summit keeps the goal in mind, but many beautiful scenes are to be observed from watching new vantage point.

You've learned that everyone wants to live on top of a mountain, but all the happiness and growth occurs whilst climbing it.

THE TREE HOUSE

Relax and allow your mind to calm down and stop unnecessary thoughts.

Image you are walking through a lovely secluded wood, slowly breathing in and out with every breath. You notice all the dead leaves on the ground and you simply love just kicking them out of the way! You realise this is childish, but who cares no one can see you as you laugh to yourself.

You are walking under a canopy of trees where you can see the sun streaming through the treetops.

You see an abundance of flowers and trees and you love being outdoors, so you find this short walk delightful. It is a lovely warm spring day and the trees are just starting to bud and showing the first signs of green. You see rich wild grasses and meadow flowers. As you walk further and further into the wood you discover an old treehouse. You just can't believe your eyes. It looks so fantastic and you wonder how long it has been here and who built it. It still looks very sturdy and strong.

You ponder for a few seconds and wonder whether you should or dare climb up it. You decide to pluck up courage and give it a go, after all nobody can see you. You gingerly try the first step and it feels quite safe and secure. You try the second and third step and it still feels strong and secure so you continue to climb up to the very top of this lovely old treehouse. When you finally reach the top, the views are fantastic and you can see all over the wood and many shorter trees and bushes. What a sight and you love being so high up too!

You decide to have a good look around the treehouse. There isn't much in it just a floor and a wooden roof. You absolutely love it. It feels like being in a fairy tale. This idyllic room is hidden away in the wood.

You forget about your worries and anxieties. There are no computers here and no television here or phones. It's all about nature.

You sit on the floor of this beautiful treehouse and take in the view. To be so high up in the trees and a long way from the ground too.

You decide to keep very still and quiet so that no wildlife or birds can see or hear you. You see a Red deer run straight underneath you and he doesn't see you at all! Another couple follow him through.

You feel invisible and it fabulous! You feel so privileged to be able to see all these animals so close to you and they don't even know you are there. You see little mice scurrying around. The lovely singing birds keep landing on the branches around you. They are so close that you could almost reach out to them and touch them. You can hear bees buzzing around everywhere.

How lovely it would be to live here all the time. No one to bother you and all our worries gone. It would be such a delightful but simple life.

Just as you decide you had better get down from the treehouse an owl, a white barn owl comes swooping down straight passed you. You find this unbelievable and so unusual to see during the day. It must have seen the mice.

You very slowly come down the steps of the treehouse and you feel so refreshed and relaxed.

What a fantastic experience for you and you certainly didn't expect to see an old abandoned treehouse on your walk through the wood.

You decide to walk back through all the trees and flowers. You come out of the wood feeling quite uplifted and so privileged.

A HOUSE IN THE WOOD, IT SEEMS LIKE A FAIRY TAIL,
BUT AT LEAST IT WASN'T MADE OF GINGERBREAD!

THE RAINBOW

Make yourself really comfortable either in your bed or in a comfy chair. Rest your head back gently so that you can read this book. Breathe deeply and relax.

This is a short relaxation meditation, one that you can use in the day when you just need 5 mins to yourself to calm down.

I want you to see and imagine in your mind a beautiful rainbow. Rainbows are perhaps the closest thing to magic! They just appear like ghostly apparitions in the sky. As the rain clears and the sun peeks out.

Every time we see a rainbow we gasp at its beauty. Adults and children alike point at it, and my word they make you feel so happy!

You are looking at this stunning rainbow and it puts you in mind of your childhood when we all believed there was a pot of gold at the end of it. That thought makes your face light up and you smile. You are looking at all the shades of the rainbow. Shades of red and orange, yellow and green, blue and indigo and not forgetting beautiful violet. Fill your mind with all these lovely colours, put everything else out of your mind and just concentrate on the now. Don't think of tomorrow or next week. Just this very special moment in time.

It is hard to imagine that this fascinating colourful arch with all its colourful beauty is caused by a combination of sunlight and rain.

Try to imagine the light rain gently falling around you and the sunlight just peeking through the clouds. What a spectacular sight and one that has us running to our windows every time that this happens.

You don't need that pot of gold to help your deepening financial crises or broken-down marriage, or the loss of someone. You can work it out for yourself and become strong. If you allow your mind to strengthen and to believe in yourself as a beautiful and intelligent clever kind person.

You are not a child anymore and you learn that there is no pot of gold at the end of the rainbow. Like most things in life every situation has its ups and downs.
Even that lovely rainbow, if you want to see the rainbow then you have to put up with the rain!

Rainbows introduce us to reflections of different beautiful possibilities, so we never forget that pain and grief are not the final option in life.
Try to be that rainbow in the storms of life.
Be the beautiful beam that smiles the day away. You love this rainbow and reminds you that even after the darkest clouds and the fiercest winds there is still beauty!
You can feel like you have all the problems on your shoulders, shrug your shoulders and release them, try to pace yourself and take things much slower if you can.
There will always be beauty in this world and in your life!

Lesley Graham

A RAINBOW IS AN ANGELS SMILE

Everybody wants happiness,
Nobody wants pain,
But you can't have a rainbow,
Without a little rain.

THE DOLPHINS

Get yourself comfortable and get ready to enjoy this lovely guided meditation.

I want you imagine that you are swimming with dolphins!

Without a doubt, there are experiences in life that prove to be unforgettable and swimming with dolphins is definitely one of them.

Imagine you are in the warmest of seas feeling so relaxed and have escaped from your anxieties back home. You are surrounded by the most gentle and loving creatures on the earth. I want you think about the powerful emotions that you experience when you are so connected to nature. They are bringing you such happiness and entertainment.

You feel such an affinity with these lovely animals, and feel that you have many characteristics that you share with them. You feel that they are having such a positive effect on you. You can feel your worries and anxiety float away. You are aware of their lovely voices and feel the healing from them, and you love the interaction with them.

You find yourself completed surrounded by them and you are right in the middle of these amazing creatures! You feel like your mind and body is being healed. It feels so positive.

Every time you have a worrying thought or your mind keeps coming back to your problems just place them on the dolphins back and let her swim away with them. Do this every time your mind wonders.

They swirl all around you generating a lot of energy and movement. This combined with such beautiful clear warm water adds to the healing. You can't help but laugh and smile constantly. Feel the happiness radiating from your body. Feel the healing. The next thing you notice is that the dolphin puts its snout on your cheek and kisses you! Such an experience for you. He comes and puts his pectoral fins around you and gives you are hug. The dolphins are creating a lot of movement in the water and the sea swirls all around you.

Don't forget if you have a thought or worry just pass it on to one of the dolphins and let them swim off with it far away and release it.
You are becoming more and more relaxed now and can imagine this scene so well. The Dolphin has very soft and rubbery skin, and you notice how they love to touch you and they also like to rub and touch each other. They are so affectionate. You have never felt anything so relaxing before and feel healed and well balanced in your mind.

You stand and watch these amazing animals for a long time and become aware of how they swim through the water. The shape of the dolphin is shaped like a tube and is pointed at both ends. They swim very fast and can swim over 20 miles per hour.

They are ducking and diving all around you and you absolutely love this experience. The effect on your body is incredible. You feel at peace with them. You also feel at peace with the world.

You look all around you and see lots of other people with dolphins all around them. You see a little boy in a wheelchair and he is laughing so much and looks so happy. You soon realise that this aquatic therapy definitely has a therapeutic effect on people with varying type of disability. People in wheelchairs have this freedom from being in the water otherwise not experienced.

You turn around once more and walk a little further in the water and notice beautiful tropical fish under the sea. The water is fairly shallow and you are so close to them and you can see them so well. The dolphins surround you again, they are kissing your cheek and hugging you and even gave you a dolphin handshake. They allow you to caress them whilst standing in knee deep clear water.

You have had an absolutely wonderful time today interacting with these highly intelligent marine mammals and you feel so much better for it. With all the warm waters of the sea and the healing that you have felt from the dolphins, it has given you the most uplifting experience.

Your worries have gone, your anxieties have gone and your mind is clear.

IF YOU CAN BELIEVE THEN YOU CAN ACHIEVE.